# COVID-19 Poetry

## *A COLLECTION OF POETIC RHYMES ~ IN COVID TIMES*

J. Michael Orr

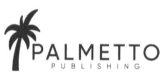

Charleston, SC
www.PalmettoPublishing.com

COVID-19 POETRY
*POETIC RHYMES ~ IN COVID TIMES*
Copyright © 2022 by J. Michael Orr

napavalleytour@sbcglobal.net

First Edition

Printed in the United States

Paperback ISBN: 978-1-68515-837-8
eBook ISBN: 978-1-68515-838-5

# *CONTENTS*

Foreword · · · · · · · · · · · · · · · · · · · · · · · · · · · · · · · vii
About the Author · · · · · · · · · · · · · · · · · · · · · · · · · viii
Introduction · · · · · · · · · · · · · · · · · · · · · · · · · · · · · ix
Prelude · · · · · · · · · · · · · · · · · · · · · · · · · · · · · · · · x

**COVID-19 PANDEMIC** · · · · · · · · · · · · · · · · · · · · 1
The visitor · · · · · · · · · · · · · · · · · · · · · · · · · · · · · · 2
To market · · · · · · · · · · · · · · · · · · · · · · · · · · · · · · · 3
Easy "Flex Pay" · · · · · · · · · · · · · · · · · · · · · · · · · · 4
No bingo · · · · · · · · · · · · · · · · · · · · · · · · · · · · · · · · 5
In my backyard · · · · · · · · · · · · · · · · · · · · · · · · · · · 6
On deaf ears fall · · · · · · · · · · · · · · · · · · · · · · · · · · 7
Such blinded eyes · · · · · · · · · · · · · · · · · · · · · · · · · 8
At journeys end · · · · · · · · · · · · · · · · · · · · · · · · · · · 9
On borrowed time · · · · · · · · · · · · · · · · · · · · · · · · · 10
At Heaven's Gate · · · · · · · · · · · · · · · · · · · · · · · · · · 11
Hope from above · · · · · · · · · · · · · · · · · · · · · · · · · · 12
Shopper or robber · · · · · · · · · · · · · · · · · · · · · · · · · 13
A COVID Relic · · · · · · · · · · · · · · · · · · · · · · · · · · · 14
Ready for the news at five · · · · · · · · · · · · · · · · · · · 15
Sorry, no vaccine yet · · · · · · · · · · · · · · · · · · · · · · · 16
His name was Chuck · · · · · · · · · · · · · · · · · · · · · · · 17
December 5 · · · · · · · · · · · · · · · · · · · · · · · · · · · · · · 18
Mother dear · · · · · · · · · · · · · · · · · · · · · · · · · · · · · · 19
"Sir, you don't look old" · · · · · · · · · · · · · · · · · · · · · 20
Shattered dreams · · · · · · · · · · · · · · · · · · · · · · · · · · 21
In outer space · · · · · · · · · · · · · · · · · · · · · · · · · · · · 22
5000 Cutouts · · · · · · · · · · · · · · · · · · · · · · · · · · · · 23
News from the UK · · · · · · · · · · · · · · · · · · · · · · · · · 24
New guy on the block · · · · · · · · · · · · · · · · · · · · · · · 25

Then comes a knock upon my door · · · · · · · · · · · · · · · · 26
Our Castle gone · · · · · · · · · · · · · · · · · · · · · · · · · · · 27
The light at tunnels end · · · · · · · · · · · · · · · · · · · · · 28
Where is our Joe? · · · · · · · · · · · · · · · · · · · · · · · · · 29
A servants tear · · · · · · · · · · · · · · · · · · · · · · · · · · · 30
Masks for thee, but not for me · · · · · · · · · · · · · · · · 31
New pills on the way · · · · · · · · · · · · · · · · · · · · · · 32
King Fauci says · · · · · · · · · · · · · · · · · · · · · · · · · · · 33

**POLITICS** · · · · · · · · · · · · · · · · · · · · · · · · · · · · · · · · **35**
The "Big Show" · · · · · · · · · · · · · · · · · · · · · · · · · · · 36
Who shall I choose? · · · · · · · · · · · · · · · · · · · · · · · 37
Down primrose path · · · · · · · · · · · · · · · · · · · · · · · 38
When time to vote · · · · · · · · · · · · · · · · · · · · · · · · · 39
The same old drip · · · · · · · · · · · · · · · · · · · · · · · · · 40
Panda poo · · · · · · · · · · · · · · · · · · · · · · · · · · · · · · · 41

**PROTESTS / DEMONSTRATIONS** · · · · · · · · · · · · · · · · · · **43**
My HOA's they clearly state · · · · · · · · · · · · · · · · · · 44
Freedoms fading light · · · · · · · · · · · · · · · · · · · · · · 45
Entitled · · · · · · · · · · · · · · · · · · · · · · · · · · · · · · · · · 46
The Naked City · · · · · · · · · · · · · · · · · · · · · · · · · · · 47
The speech · · · · · · · · · · · · · · · · · · · · · · · · · · · · · · 48
So safe within · · · · · · · · · · · · · · · · · · · · · · · · · · · · 49
Down hallowed halls · · · · · · · · · · · · · · · · · · · · · · · 50
Strike up the band! · · · · · · · · · · · · · · · · · · · · · · · · 51
Little girls and little boys · · · · · · · · · · · · · · · · · · · · 52
Those statues must come down · · · · · · · · · · · · · · · · 53
The "Narrow" Gate · · · · · · · · · · · · · · · · · · · · · · · · 54
Our small cabin · · · · · · · · · · · · · · · · · · · · · · · · · · · 55
Our hallowed flag · · · · · · · · · · · · · · · · · · · · · · · · · 56
Roaming dogs · · · · · · · · · · · · · · · · · · · · · · · · · · · · 57
The Dumpty falls · · · · · · · · · · · · · · · · · · · · · · · · · 58

Lest we should faint · · · · · · · · · · · · · · · · · · · · · 59
Old Pete · · · · · · · · · · · · · · · · · · · · · · · · · · 60
The Declaration · · · · · · · · · · · · · · · · · · · · · · 61
I was only eight · · · · · · · · · · · · · · · · · · · · · · 62
While on the beat · · · · · · · · · · · · · · · · · · · · · 63

**KENOSHA** · · · · · · · · · · · · · · · · · · · · · · · **65**
Kenosha Kyle · · · · · · · · · · · · · · · · · · · · · · · 66

**MEXICO BORDER CRISIS** · · · · · · · · · · · · · · **67**
No need to fret · · · · · · · · · · · · · · · · · · · · · · 68
Oh sleepy Joe · · · · · · · · · · · · · · · · · · · · · · · 69
"Come on man!" · · · · · · · · · · · · · · · · · · · · · · 70

**AFGHANISTAN WITHDRAWAL** · · · · · · · · · · **71**
It's just my style · · · · · · · · · · · · · · · · · · · · · 72
Coffins off the plane · · · · · · · · · · · · · · · · · · · 73

**HOMELESSNESS** · · · · · · · · · · · · · · · · · · · **75**
"Un"Golden Gate · · · · · · · · · · · · · · · · · · · · · 76

**CANCEL CULTURE** · · · · · · · · · · · · · · · · · · **77**
Just a myth · · · · · · · · · · · · · · · · · · · · · · · · 78
Two farts only ~ The "New Code" · · · · · · · · · · · 79

**MISS "MURDER HORNET"** · · · · · · · · · · · · · **81**
What is her name? · · · · · · · · · · · · · · · · · · · · 82
"What the hell is that!" · · · · · · · · · · · · · · · · · 83

**CALIFORNIA** · · · · · · · · · · · · · · · · · · · · · **85**
"EAST we go" · · · · · · · · · · · · · · · · · · · · · · · 86
California ash · · · · · · · · · · · · · · · · · · · · · · · 87
California Oil Spill - October 1, 2021 · · · · · · · · · 88

**EVERYDAY STUFF** · · · · · · · · · · · · · · · · · · · · · · · · · **89**
You are caller 9 · · · · · · · · · · · · · · · · · · · · · · · · · · 90

**OLD AGE** · · · · · · · · · · · · · · · · · · · · · · · · · · · · · **91**
Mind go, body no · · · · · · · · · · · · · · · · · · · · · · · 92
I've now got to pee! · · · · · · · · · · · · · · · · · · · · · 93
Six times a night · · · · · · · · · · · · · · · · · · · · · · · 94
Don't want to fall · · · · · · · · · · · · · · · · · · · · · · 95
Someday you'll know · · · · · · · · · · · · · · · · · · · · 96
Lost brother dear · · · · · · · · · · · · · · · · · · · · · · · 97
The place I knew · · · · · · · · · · · · · · · · · · · · · · · 98

**THE FINAL RHYME** · · · · · · · · · · · · · · · · · · · · · **99**
81 rhymes I did write · · · · · · · · · · · · · · · · · · · · 99

# FOREWORD

If not for the Corona virus escaping from China, many verses in this book could not have been written. Also negligent were those officials who placed elderly COVID patients in Nursing Homes with others who had not contracted the virus, resulting in thousands of deaths. Further confusion resulted from our government "flip flopping" on such matters as protective masks, the virus curve, social distancing, quarantines, closing businesses, vaccines, and other issues.

Several politicians also continued to advise us how to protect ourselves with masks and social distancing, while at the same time violating their own advice, not wearing masks and mixing with others at parties across the country. President Biden's "Open Door" policy at our southern border was also a factor. Allowing thousands of "unvaccinated" migrants into our country while at the same time mandating vaccinations for US citizens contributed to further confusion.

The greatest hero's during the pandemic were those brave Doctors, Nurses, and other medical personal across the nation who dedicated their lives to treating those with the virus, many paying the ultimate price for such devotion.

# ABOUT THE AUTHOR

J. Michael Orr was born in up-
state New York in 1940. He holds a
degree in Health Science from San
Francisco State College and attend-
ed graduate school at Golden Gate
College. A graduate of the Santa Rosa
School of Nursing, he also worked as
a Psychiatric Nurse for the California
Department of Mental Hygiene and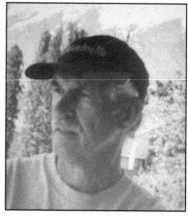
served in the Army Nurse Corp during the Vietnam War where he
met his wife Joan who was also an Army Nurse. Upon completing
military service, he left the Nursing Profession to become a Deputy
Probation Officer in the state of California, ultimately attaining an
administrative position within that field.

The author has also published two other books, *A Day or Two in
the Napa Valley*, a travel book oriented to the famous Napa Valley
California wine region, and *Rock n' Roll'n ~ The 50's and 60's*, an
autobiography about growing up during that fabulous Rock and Roll
era. He is also an accomplished artist, well known for his work in
the Napa Valley wine country. His work is extensively collected.

# *INTRODUCTION*

Back in 2019, I decided to try my hand at writing poetry. Verses in the form of "Rhymes" began spontaneously popping into my mind, so I started jotting them down. At the end of 2019, COVID-19 dropped a bomb on us all. At the time, a host of other serious matters were affecting our country well into 2020 and beyond. Throughout 2020 and 2021, I continued writing verses about COVID-19 issues plus other events as they occurred. Two and one half years later I finished the 81st, ironically my age at the time. In December of 2021, when we all thought COVID-19 was beginning to wane a bit, a new visitor called Omicron arrived one morning and decided to take up residence well into 2022.

# *PRELUDE*

Please read the narrative page preceding the rhymes in each section. This way you'll get a feel of what's coming.

The years 2020, 2021, and into 2022 had their share of riveting events. Many of the subjects noted address serious issues. However, I've also included some humor, patriotism, and other words of "hope" along the way. Finally, the "Last Rhyme," the 81st, my age at the time I finished, two and one-half years after beginning.

# COVID-19 PANDEMIC

COVID-19 paid a visit to the world in late 2019 and continued throughout 2020, 2021, and well into 2022. Millions of people died as a result. The price of it's effects included wearing masks, social distancing, quarantines, being shuttered in our homes for extended periods, plus other consequences. Many businesses closed causing thousands to lose their jobs. At times, things seemed to get better, giving people a false sense of security as they returned to the beaches and began mingling again. However, the virus returned with a vengeance. We were then told a vaccine was coming, but often received mixed messages about the vaccine, wearing masks or not wearing them, virus curve up or down, plus other confusing mandates. The vaccine finally arrived, the elderly receiving it first as they stood in long lines on cold freezing days waiting to get the jab.

Although life in many ways came to a standstill, other activities such as baseball, football and basketball continued with an interesting twist. Instead of spectators in the stands, cardboard cutouts replaced them. Loud noise was also piped in to simulate the noise of the crowd.

Much hypocrisy continued as many elected officials violated the same rules and precautions others throughout the country were expected to follow.

Back in late 2019, a stranger came knocking on our door.

## *The visitor*

This stranger came to us one day
A needless price we all would pay
Adorned with masks upon our face
Lock up the doors, shut down the place
Our thoughts and prayers, our fate unknown
The massive graves so neatly sown
A hostile foe to so contend
The question was, "When would it end?"

Although COVID-19 was rampant throughout the land, we still had to buy food and other stuff, especially toilet paper. So we put on our masks and headed out, yet afraid someone might sneeze on us in the market.

## *To market*

With mask secure, and gloves in tow
Its off to market now I go
Then finally there and in the door
To find the stuff I'm looking for
A clerk then says, "I'll help you please"
"No thanks my lad," as then I sneeze
"It's just a cold, no problem son"
Then like a rocket off he runs!
Now down my row a shopper comes
His eyes ablaze, his nose a-run
With mask secure, and gloves in tow
I quickly sprint back down my row
Crash out the door and home I go
Without the stuff I needed so!

So maybe you lost your job as a result of COVID, or you just retired looking forward to that trip you planned. Whatever the situation, our lives dramatically changed. Many of us simply stayed home and hunkered down, waiting for the next news release, or watching all the boring stuff on TV.

## *Easy "Flex Pay"*

I change the channels every day
And wait til COVID goes away
The same old stuff goes on and on
The game show hosts, the endless con
The easy "Flex Pay" can arrive
As now the market takes a dive
This chair keeps making my butt sore
I'm sick of this, can't take no more!

Back in the summer of 2019, you may have enjoyed a weekly bingo game, or getting together with friends down at the local pub, or planning a winter trip someplace. Then in late 2019, because of an error by some clucks over in a place called Wuhan, China, this toxic bug got loose and affected us all, some more than others.

## *No bingo*

This cabin fever really sucks
All brought about by Wuhan clucks
Must stay inside and cannot go
Down to my favorite movie show
Now in the wings such tragedy
With signs out front, "No Vacancy"
And on and on throughout the night
With steadfast effort as they fight
A team that stands to meet the task
So tightly fit with gown and mask
Then in the air we finally see
A flattened curve, such blissful glee
But my State says I cannot go
No job…No life…now no bingo

We all need a special place where we can go now and then for some quiet time; a place to think, rest, or pray. I like gardening and growing flowers. At my place things start blooming around late April. Maybe your place is the same, or you might live in an apartment and have a veranda or balcony you can look out from. In April of 2020, we all needed a quiet place to rest, pray, or meditate as the Corona virus wreaked havoc across our country.

# *In my backyard*

In my backyard yard a moment take
To wait the flowers bloom to make
This quarantine may someday leave
But as for now I make believe
I'm on an island distant calm
With ocean breeze, and swaying palm
It's said a vaccine soon may come
To free us from this maelstrom
But as for now I sit alone
While God's sweet comfort from his throne
Does help me through this trial again
As in the past…my trusted friend

*"You are my hiding place; you will protect me from trouble and surround me with songs of deliverance."*

Psalm 32:7

As a result of COVID-19, some Governors shut down businesses completely in their state, causing thousands to lose their jobs. Maybe you were one of those who marched to your state capitol to protest and present your case.

## *On deaf ears fall*

At Governor's gate we did arrive
To plead our case, to stay alive
"We've got your backs, no need to care"
"It's for your good," our Gov's declare
"But sir you don't quite understand"
"My wife, my child…this wasn't planned"
Our fervent cry, our desperate call
Our pleas alas on deaf ears fall
"But sir, you still don't understand"
"My wife, my child…this wasn't planned"

Despite warnings from our Government and the Center for Disease Control, throngs of people flocked to beaches across the country in the summer of 2020.

## Such blinded eyes

The beach crowds back with such delight
Believing things were then all right
The hair salons and barber shops
Concession stands and lollipops
But hid within a boardwalk crack
While planning a new sneak attack
A cunning foe with army strong
Peered with delight at beaches throng
Then struck again to such surprise
At huddled mass…such blinded eyes

COVID affected all of us one way or another. Before it arrived in late 2019, we had our dreams, our plans, our goals. For most, the virus made things difficult in our lives. For others, the ultimate price would be paid.

## *At journeys end*

So up the mountain I did climb
The sun above did brightly shine
On treasure that was clear in sight
As darkness then brought on the night
This thief he came from far away
A heavy price I was to pay
Such wretched foe within his grip
As waves upon a sinking ship
Awake and faint I realize
At journey's end…to my surprise

The elderly were most affected by the virus, especially those with underlying conditions. Yet, many survived, only to be visited by another villain.

## *On borrowed time*

Corona seems to be in past
It's horrid spikes not long would last
To clamp upon our breath so tight
At reapers door throughout the night
But now we relics have survived
On borrowed time to stay alive
Then comes a new knock on the door
This deviant not bargained for
So now I guess the best we can
Is trust in God, not fellow man
To hope and ever steadfast pray
For strength to last another day

*"Many are the afflictions of the righteous, but the LORD delivers him from them all"*

Psalm 34:19

Many affected by the virus placed their faith and trust in God, knowing a room and bed had already been reserved for them beyond Heaven's Gate.

## *At Heaven's Gate*

Though body tired, and future dim
My hope doth lie past Earthly rim
Above the sky to soon apply
The key that's made for not to die
A room and bed that now is made
Beyond this life's confused parade
The joy for me that now does wait
So patiently…at Heaven's Gate

*"And God shall wipe away all tears from their eyes; and there shall be no more death, neither sorrow, nor crying, neither shall there be any more pain: for the former things are passed away."*

Revelation 21:4

COVID continued its grip throughout 2020, 2021, well into 2022. The virus "curve" vacillated up and down. A false sense of hope continued to be presented by the government, yet many found little solace in such promises, turning instead to God in the midst of the continuing tribulation.

## *Hope from above*

Will this dilemma ever cease
As COVID's grip to yet release
The curve it seems to give us hope
Yet in our lives this slippery slope
Continues as we strive to live
From day to day a narrative
That spans the broad variety
From happiness to lethargy
And now again the sun does rise
On broken hearts and tearful eyes
The hope that can but only come
From God above…from his kingdom

*"Through the Lord's mercies we are not consumed, because His compassions fail not"*

Lamentations 3:22

Back in the days of the "old west" thieves and villains who robbed banks, trains, and stagecoaches would often wear "Masks" to conceal their identity. Ironically, because of mask mandates instituted throughout the COVID pandemic, you couldn't distinguish the good guys from the bad!

## *Shopper or robber*

While shopping late the other night
As I did have my mask on tight
This shadow entered by the door
With mask adorned into the store
It then slipped down the dim lit rows
But chose no goods, as normal goes
Then came this thought within my mind
As shadow came up close behind
Was it there just to shop for tea
Or was it there to rob from me?

When you're very old, at times such things as COVID, Delta Variant, and Omicron don't seem to matter much. You're already overweight, have a heart problem, and take blood thinners. One step on a banana peel and that's it! Your primary goal is to simply enjoy the day and with any luck make it to the next!

## *A COVID Relic*

I wash my hands and wear my mask
And try my best to meet the task
But what the hell, I'm 91
Forget it man, just want some fun!
The TV shows are such a bore
And I'm so old, don't care no more
I sit around and scratch my butt
While looked upon as old fart nut
A remnant of a bygone age
To place inside the relics cage
So bring the pie and ice cream bowl
The bacon fat to soothe my soul
But now I'm told to lose some weight
That chocolate cake…it sure looks great!

More confusion continued throughout the COVID pandemic, especially affecting older folks who simply wanted to make it through the day, plop down in their chair at five, watch the evening news, then hit the rack at eight!

## *Ready for the news at five*

Another day gone by its said
Too many from Corona dead
The curve still like a coaster ride
First up then down the other side
To wear a mask or not I'm told
I'm so confused and just too old
Have trouble getting out of bed
Now all of this to ache my head
So take my pills to stay alive
Get ready for the news at five
Then listen to the same old crock
Now into bed at 8 o'clock
If I should die before I wake
I pray the Lord my soul to take

Throughout 2020, we were promised a vaccine was coming to address the COVID-19 issue. Then trials of the vaccine resulted in a few adverse reactions causing delay's in the vaccine being distributed to the population.

## *Sorry, no vaccine yet*

Was told the vaccine soon would tell
If trials were going very well
Then some reactions did occur
Now everything seems such a blur
Was counting so upon that shot
And thought that it would quickly blot
This horrid nightmare from my life
And also help my anxious wife
Who says she's sick and tired of
Still waiting for help from above
So here we sit and place our bet
Yet now we're told…no vaccine yet!

Many of us either got the virus or knew those who were affected by it. Sadly, we may have known someone who succumbed to it. In late 2019, just before COVID began spreading throughout the country, I attended an event in my hometown. During the event, a guy I knew from High School approached me.

## *His name was Chuck*

At shindig of the old and gray
This guy came up to me one day
"Hey Jim, I'm Chuck" he did proclaim
"Remember me, recall my name?"
"Why yes, I do remember you"
"We're still alive, but very few"
So talked awhile and did recall
Our younger days when we stood tall
Then many months one day did come
A letter and a comment from
His wife who said that Chuck had gone
A COVID loss…one early dawn

I wrote this rhyme on December 5, 2021, praying to make it to December 6. Had my two vaccine jabs and my "booster" shot, so figured everything was OK. Then we heard many who were vaccinated were getting the virus anyway. This COVID-19 guy never gives up! Your cat is supposed to have 9 lives. Maybe there's a reason this cat is called COVID….19!

# December 5

December 5 and still alive
Corona here did not arrive
But out there lurking someplace yet
To pounce on me lest I forget
The scourge that's taken many souls
Still on the highway it patrols
This toxic villain wants to creep
And catch me napping at my sleep
So must avoid his fancy tricks
If I desire December 6
So shut the gate that opens wide
And not allow this cat inside
I must take care for goodness sake
Lest COVID guy… my life will take!

We all had friends, relatives, mothers, fathers, or grandparents who were afflicted with the virus. Some needed to be hospitalized. Sadly, because of the virulent and contagious nature of the virus, we were restricted from visiting our loved ones.

## *Mother dear*

I pray the time will come someday
When back we'll look and maybe say
All this was for the better good
While in long lines so many stood
To take their test or get their shot
That may just help, or maybe not
Now mother dear in nursing bed
So ill from this Corona dread
And her I'm told I cannot see
A victim maybe I could be
So here I sit in deep despair
And send to God another prayer

The elderly were more susceptible to the effects of the virus. It was decided they should receive the vaccine first. So they stood in lines on cold winter days to get it. However, keeping with the often vile nature of the species, many "younger" citizens dressed up in old tattered clothing in an effort to give the appearance of being old, then snuck into the same lines. Had to get their jab too right?

## *"Sir, you don't look old"*

I'm standing here to get my shot
The COVID fix or maybe not
They said because I'm 83
Could get in line they'd give to me
So here I stand in bitter cold
But guy up front don't look that old
All dressed in granny outfit nice
While waiting here on frozen ice
So asked him,"Hey, you don't look old?"
As he replied with words so bold
"For what its worth I'm 33"
"This granny outfit gave to me"
"By my sweet Grandma she did say"
"Get in that line… or price you'll pay!"

Having worked so hard to fulfill their dreams, some found them shattered on the rocks as COVID took its toll. Sadly, many lives were lost, many relationships severed.

## *Shattered dreams*

The plans we made, our dreams so clear
Brought such content as they drew near
We strained and toiled to meet the goals
As those before, our dear lost souls
We shut the gate, and locked the door
So safe inside for evermore
The sunlight did so brightly shine
On our domain, both yours and mine
Then COVID did arrive one day
And took the one I thought would stay
Our shattered dreams, this empty life
The lonely days without my wife

So there were these wealthy folks who built a rocket ship and went up into outer space for a few minutes. They all floated around weightless in their capsule, but wore no masks?

## *In outer space*

Those people up in outer space
They have no mask upon their face
Does COVID not exist up there?
Way out beyond the thin blue air?
If that is so, please sign me up
I'll get a seat and take my pup
Forget these condo owners fee's
I want a ticket…take me please!

Although life in many ways came to a standstill during the pandemic, other activities such as baseball, football and basketball continued with an interesting twist. Instead of spectators in the stands, cardboard cutouts replaced them. Loud noise was also piped in to simulate the noise of the crowd.

## *5000 Cutouts*

The fake crowd noise was piped in loud
To simulate the blaring crowd
Five thousand cutouts in the stands
Sat motionless upon their hands
They seemed confused and could not cheer
Nor even have an ice cold beer
While outside all the people wait
For some vaccine... if not too late

In 2021, a new COVID variant was found to be prevalent in the United Kingdom. Its name ~ Delta Variant.

## *News from the UK*

What is this brand new strain they say
Called Delta "V" now in UK
We thought this thing was fixed by now
As comes more sweat upon our brow
This COVID guy he's such a brat
So many lives like my sweet cat
But even little kittens may
Scratch deep and often make you pay
So now we wait to get the shot
Then back to normal….maybe not

So I got my shots, got my booster, now everything seemed OK. I can now take my mask off and head down to the pub to have a few brews with the guys. Right?

## *New guy on the block*

The vaccine shot it made me glad
Now I can be a happy lad
With no more mask and itchy face
Put on my hat and quickly race
Down to the pub with friends I knew
To shoot some dice and have a few
Then TV blares upon the wall
A newsflash comes for one and all
"Look out for new guy on the block!"
"He's armed and wants to clean your clock"
So what's his name, and who is he?
"I think they call him…Delta V"

Having had many close calls with the Grim Reaper, I know what its like to be in a hospital bed not knowing whether I might live to see another day. Maybe you've had a similar experience.

## *Then comes a knock upon my door*

What is this scourge upon me so
With aching frame that cannot go
As morning dawns again once more
The stage now set, my body sore
I look upon the window glass
And see myself as withered grass
All faded and no more can stand
Like house upon the sinking sand
Then comes a knock upon my door

Prior to COVID, across the land there were those who were either building a home, establishing a new business, making plans, whatever. Then suddenly an uninvited guest arrived to rob them.

## *Our Castle gone*

Corona came and hurt us so
The things we built did quickly go
Our Castle took so long to make
Now stands alone, no care to take
The days and nights, the toil and sweat
The stately yard, the B-Ball net
Our flower bed now jungle scrub
No parties at the Country Club
Corona came and hurt us so
The things we built, did quickly go

We were told, "There's light at the end of the tunnel" while we rode the train of promises as COVID continued taking its toll. Then a new surprise!

## The light at tunnels end

This journey seems so very long
As COVID one day came along
To strike at us already frail
Despite our fight to no avail
The ride we're told would someday end
As we continued to descend
Into this deep and dark abyss
Our fears the experts did dismiss
As foolish naive childish thoughts
From weak and blinded tiny tots
Yet then we saw around the bend
A light at tunnels final end
An answer to our labored plight?
At journeys end throughout the night?
But then an utter stark surprise
As light did blind our weakened eyes
The light at very tunnels end
Was really not our foretold friend
A new and unexpected slant
*"Hello...I'm Delta Variant"*

President Joe Biden promised COVID would go away quickly. It didn't. He also promised unity and prosperity. That didn't happen. Instead we got chaos and inflation. He didn't have the usual press conferences either, and seemed to "hide out" on occasion. When he did come to the podium, he looked tired and often seemed confused.

## *Where is our Joe?*

Corona thing won't go away
Now Delta "V" seems here to stay
Put masks back on now is the rule
For kids in even Sunday school
With Afghan's heading for the door
And Taliban now in the store
Here comes this new brat in the place
Its Omicron now in our face
So where's our Joe...not on the map?
Don't bother him...he needs his nap!

Is this what that man may have felt, upon the cross as woman knelt.

## *A servants tear*

Corona came to me one day
A heavy price was asked to pay
I lie awake all through the night
As pain and anguish gripped me tight
Is this what that man may have felt?
Upon the cross as woman knelt
Before him as his blood did flow
Down weakened body ever slow
Is this what maybe he did feel?
This pain and anguish as I kneel
Before him now that he might hear
My prayer and heal a servants tear


*"The afflictions of the righteous are many, but the Lord delivers him from them all"*

Psalm 34:19

Much hypocrisy continued during the COVID pandemic as many elected officials violated the same rules we were all ordered to follow.

## *Masks for thee, but not for me*

The Napa Valley it's so nice
With Newsom's crowd, champagne on ice
While at French Laundry with his crew
No masks on Gavin's fine menu
They don't need masks, its plain to see
If not for them, then why for me?
How come this rule that I must wear?
What's up with that?... It just ain't fair!
Now Nancy's gang up there to play
No masks for her, just Chardonnay
These hypocrites do so decree
"Its masks for thee...but not for me"

Easy-to-take antiviral pills were hailed as a potential turning point in the fight against the coronavirus because of the medicines ability to keep high-risk people out of the hospital. But doctors reported the limited supply of the pills meant they were unlikely to alleviate the strain on many hospitals confronting climbing admissions and staffing shortages made worse by Omicron infections. Many continued to be frustrated and simply gave up hope.

## New pills on the way

They say the vaccine it may fix
But if it don't, more pills in mix
Some brand new drugs now on the way
But heavy price may need to pay
I'm tired of all this stuff you see
Who cares, so what, no more for me!

Dr. Anthony Fauci was the Director of the National Institute of Allergy and Infectious Diseases & White House Chief Medical Advisor. We all saw him on TV from time to time giving us advice on masks, vaccines, virus curve up or down, and more. Often, his advice and conclusions appeared to be confusing and inaccurate.

## *King Fauci says*

King Fauci he does now declare
You must wear your mask everywhere
"Oh mighty King then I must ask"
"In my own bathroom wear my mask?"
"Why yes my child, you should take care"
"You never know who may be there"
"But must I wear my mask to bed?"
"I think you should"… King Fauci said

# *POLITICS*

Politics also shared the stage during 2020, 2021, and into 2022. The Presidential debate took place on September 29, 2020, a ten round brawl between incumbent Donald Trump and challenger Joe Biden. Moderator Chris Wallace had a tough time controlling the fight. Finally, election time arrived in November, Joe Biden winning a hotly contested race.

Democrats now in control, things were going to get better. But the same old drip continued. President Joe Biden promised a new path to "Unity" and "Prosperity." Instead, we received the Afghanistan debacle, the US Border crisis, Inflation, sky high gas prices, and discourse throughout the country.

In addition, during 2020 President Joe Biden's son Hunter became the target of many, suggesting he colluded with the Chinese government for monetary favors.

Political divide continued between Republicans and Democrats as both parties struggled to initiate their agenda's.

The Presidential debate took place on September 29, 2020, a ten round brawl between incumbent Donald Trump and challenger Joe Biden.

## The "Big Show"

The "Big Debate" was quite a show
A bloody match with Don & Joe
Ten rounds of thunder on the stage
Like two crazed lions in a cage
Their handler Chris could not control
As they began to "Rock & Roll"
So next time if they start to lip
Their handler better bring a "Whip!"

In November of 2020, we had two to choose from for President of the United States, incumbent Donald Trump and contender Joe Biden.

## *Who shall I choose?*

So then we had from two to choose
The one would win, the other loose
And Don said "I'm the better man"
But Joe thought he was greater than
The one who was in White House place
Who tried his best to make the case
And scale the tall and grueling wall
Like Humpty Dumpty not to fall
So then we had from two to choose
The one would win, the other loose

Joe Biden got elected President of the United States. He promised a new path forward; unity, prosperity, harmony, and job opportunities. Come on man! Instead we got more COVID, higher gas prices, inflation, an open border, more poverty, and continued discourse within the nation.

## *Down primrose path*

Election it was finally done
The marchers finished with their fun
An old guy now to make things new
At least that's what he said he'd do
So here we go down primrose path
With barbed wire laid to stem the wrath
But Joe's been in now for sometime
My gas at pump $4.99!
Inflation rampant in the sky
And T-bone steak I cannot buy
Is this the path he chose for us?
Cause if it was…I'm off this bus!

Regarding President Joe Biden's "Open Border" policy :

## *When time to vote*

"Hey, come on man cross border wall"

"I've got your back, you'll have a ball"

"Jump on that bus right over there"

"And join your friends without a care"

"We'll take you to a nice hotel"

"And clean you up, just ring the bell"

"You have no money now you say?"

"No problem friend, no need to pay"

"But now you think you COVID ache?"

"The vaccine maybe you should take?"

"Forget it man, you'll be okay"

"Get on that bus, now don't delay"

"I've made the locals take the shot"

"So they'll be safe, if that you've got"

"Now bon voyage, be on your way"

"I've got your back, you'll be okay"

"And don't forget when time to vote"

"My name is Joe, please make a note"

I think I'll watch Flea Market Flip!

## *The same old drip*

This country's gone too far astray
As nothing makes no sense today
The bitter gall, the angry mobs
The "Peaceful" protests, looter slobs
And now debates to fix all this
With promises of tranquil bliss
It sounds like just the same old drip
I think I'll watch Flea Market Flip!

Joe Biden's son Hunter became the target of many, suggesting he colluded with the Chinese government for monetary favors. He denied this of course. Joe said he was basically a trusting soul, and also a great artist!

# *Panda poo*

"Oh Hunter, Hunter, what'd you do?"
"Did you go step in Panda Poo?"
Those Panda's love their bamboo shoot
And everyone loves extra loot
"So "Come on Man," your on a roll"
"Your Dad says you're a trusting soul"
"So keep on painting if you can"
"A lot more scratch could be at hand!"

# *PROTESTS / DEMONSTRATIONS*

On May 25, 2020, a Minneapolis, Minnesota black man, George Floyd, was murdered by police officer, Derek Chauvin. His death resulted in a rash of protests and demonstrations across the country. Some were peaceful, others violent as mobs roamed cities destroying property, looting businesses, and at times shooting police officers. On 05/28/2020, mobs burned down the 3rd precinct headquarters of the Police Department in Minneapolis. Rampant shootings and violence continued throughout 2020, 2021, and well into 2022, especially affecting African American communities. Innocent children were often victims of these violent acts.

Other protests were directed at the issue of racism. Confederate statues and other statues including those of slave traders and Christopher Columbus were toppled throughout the country. Many also questioned the validity of the Declaration of Independence, criticizing the basis of the document.

On January 6, 2021, a violent demonstration took place at the United States Capitol in Washington, DC, where a mob sought to overturn the 2020 presidential election by disrupting a joint session of Congress.

In 2020, a St. Louis Missouri couple brandished their weapons in order to protect their home from an apparent BLM protest group who had broken through a gate entrance near their property, confronting them in front of their home.

## *My HOA's they clearly state*

Whoever thought that this would come
To my nice hood so neatly run
The HOA's they clearly state
No drugs, no mobs, no demonstrate
Yet crowds and tents go on and on
With dogs unleashed, and smell so strong
So stopped this guy and asked one day
"What caused your life to such decay?"
With anger then he so replied
"It's your fault ma'am…get back inside!"

Peaceful protests fine. Mob rule and destruction not fine! Throughout our country during 2020 and 2021, mob rule manifested itself in major metropolitan cities.

## *Freedoms fading light*

Our country no more like it was
In days gone by and this because
Of frenzied mobs, and disrespect
With riots, looting, families wrecked
As protests spread across the land
The multitude of rabbles band
Together decked in hoodies shroud
To make their point so blaring loud
With such deceit and brick in hand
They ravage this our beauty land
To take away forefathers fight
That so established freedoms light

In places such as Minneapolis, Minnesota and Kenosha, Wisconsin, hoodlums and thugs turned what may have begun as "Peaceful Protests" into wild savage orgy's where businesses were destroyed and looted. In most cases nothing was done to bring the perpetrators to justice.

## *Entitled*

Now comes this madness to our land
It shakes the Devil's evil hand
As masses gather to destroy
The things that others do employ
The looters, thugs, and wild mob
Who feel entitled as they rob
From those who've labored oh so hard
Now find their lives so deeply scarred
Then comes this Dapper Dan so neat
Who struts down city's broken street
He looks so fine, and clothed so well
A bonus from his vast pell-mell

As many were aware, on May 25, 2020, a Minneapolis, Minnesota black man, George Floyd, was murdered by police officer, Derek Chauvin, resulting in a rash of violent protests. Violent mobs roamed cities destroying property, looting businesses, and at times shooting police officers. On 05/28/2020, mobs burned down the 3rd precinct headquarters of the Police Department in Minneapolis.

## *The Naked City*

From round the country came them all
To Minneapolis and St.Paul
For George with voices ever loud
This wild and angry rabid crowd
All laced with hatred and despise
With rage and malice in their eyes
Such vulgar lingo they did whine
At those along the thin blue line
With fire and brimstone they did say
"Burn down 3rd precinct price to pay!"
"Five miles of Lake Street we'll destroy"
"With rocks and bottles to employ"
Then after mayhem where were they?
These "peaceful" crowds that came to play?
Back in their holes they all did run
To lurk again… until more fun

Some of us may have had the unfortunate experience of being stopped in traffic during a protest on a major freeway. Frustrated and unable to get to work on time, we may have attempted to get through in whatever manner we could.

# *The speech*

Now eggs for breakfast, coffee too
I'm out the door, down avenue
The traffic stopped "Protest Today"
"Who has the right to block my way?"
Then comes these two from other side
These brats who wish to block my ride
Upon my hood they scream and scoff
As I speed up, they both fall off
Now at the office in I go
To make my speech and extra dough
But then one dressed in sparkling blue
Comes in the room to ask a few
"Recall those two fell off your hood?"
"Why yes I do, as best I could"
"But what does this to do with me?"
"Please come with me, one died you see"

Demonstrations and protests continued throughout 2020, 2021, and 2022. Residents often felt threatened as groups of marchers passed by their homes and businesses, reminded of the destruction and damage that occurred during the riots in many metropolitan cities.

## *So safe within*

The days of wine and roses gone
As thoughts uncertain ever spawn
Within our hearts and minds so clear
While protest marchers come to cheer
But safe within we occupy
As echelons of ruin pass by
Yet still we do quite often fear
This rebel band as it comes near

On January 6, 2021, a violent demonstration took place at the United States Capitol in Washington, DC where a mob sought to overturn the 2020 presidential election by disrupting a joint session of Congress.

## *Down hallowed halls*

The days of troubled times and pain
As angered crowds with fury reign
Across the land to country's den
Red, White, and Blue these angry men
And woman too with flags held high
Did storm the house with maddened cry
Such rage at stolen choice they say
Did so occur election day
So what about this endless clatter?
And what conclusion of the matter?
Fear God and keep his sacred word
Should be the duty of the herd
For in the end all deeds will lay
At God's pure throne, lest all should pray

More on the January 6, 2021, violent demonstration that took place at the United States Capitol in Washington, DC.

## *Strike up the band!*

Such fog and vast uncertainty
A veil that shrouds humanity
The masses stormed the Citadel
With flags and banners as they fell
Upon the hallowed marble floors
As others stormed the Senate doors
To enter in and take command
"We've got control, strike up the band!"
But some with honor there sincere
While others just to smoke and cheer
What was the end of this demise?
A barbed wire fence… to our surprise?

Many protests and demonstrations during 2020 and 2021 were directed at the issue of racism. Acts of vandalism supporting this position included the toppling of monuments such as Confederate statues, statues apparently seen as representing slave traders, and a statue of Christopher Columbus.

## *Little girls and little boys*

See little children how they run
To tear down statues just for fun
These little girls and little boys
As if destroying all their toys
To think it such a noble cause
Not taking time to simply pause
And ponder all the many scars
While looking through the jail house bars
"Oh Mommy, Daddy...where are you?"
"Am I not of the chosen few?"

"I'm not sure I understand your position on why you feel ALL statues must be torn down. Can you clarify it a bit more?"

## *Those statues must come down*

"You've got the answer you do say"

"You sure you haven't gone astray?"

"You say your path it seems so right"

"To get this country back in sight"

"In sight of what if you don't mind?"

"What is your case still undefined?"

"Well first those statues must come down"

"They represent not black or brown"

"Oh now I get it very clear"

"With statues gone, you have no fear"

"Well that's not the entire case"

"To satisfy our oppressed race"

"Then what else is it you require?"

"We'd like much more... that's our desire"

More statues fell during 2020 and 2021. Protestors continued to declare, "Our way is right because it's new!" "Your leaders know not what they do!" In the bedlam, behind a "Narrow Gate" a voice beckoned.

## The "Narrow" Gate

Like birth pains at the very end
The monuments did quickly bend
Like Humpty Dumpty on the wall
The statues round us they did fall
Torn down by children in the fog
Whose loud and railing dialogue
Consumed the airways day by day
With rage and anger they did say
"Our way is right because it's new!"
"Your leaders know not what they do!"
Yet in the bedlam some did see
A "Narrow Gate" that beckoned thee
"Please open up and look behind"
As came this voice so pure and kind
That struck at hearts like sharpened knife
"I am the way, the truth, the life"

Some angry protestor's felt they were "Entitled" to the possessions others had worked so hard for all their lives, especially their homes!

## *Our small cabin*

I had a dream the other night
As storm clouds filled the sky with fright
The crowds of angry souls pressed in
To terrorize our small cabin
Where I had lived so very long
With wife and dog as angry throng
At doorstep did they so decree
"Your cabin now is ours you see,"
"So pack your bags, you now must leave!"
"No time for you or wife to grieve"
But yield not as I did load
My 38 that could explode
"Please say hello to Smith & Wesson"
"You're now about to learn a lesson!"

Many senseless protestors exercised their First Amendment right at times, burning and destroying the flag of the United States of America, forgetful of the blood and sacrifice paid by others that gave them the right to disparage such a treasured gift.

## *Our hallowed flag*

The Red, the White, and then the Blue
A country founded just for you
A privilege you received at birth
No other place so free on earth
But in your selfish childish way
Would see the colors no more sway
From freedoms palette vivid shown
For selfish reasons of your own
Lest you forget, or may not know
Was young men's blood shed long ago
On distant shores and baron lands
Who gave their lives on island sands
So you could live and not destroy
The many fruits you now enjoy
So listen friend to this advise
It was for you…your freedom's price

Although many demonstrations were peaceful in 2020 and 2021, others turned violent as mobs of hoodlums roamed the streets of many metropolitan cities. Often, with no regard for their actions, these mobs looted and destroyed local mom and pop businesses operated by simple law abiding citizens.

## *Roaming dogs*

The mobs continued to destroy
Such evil methods they employ
A force that pains the simple man
Whose business gone by caravan
Of roaming dogs with vile disgust
To feed their wicked hateful lust
What should their end thus made to be
A long confined reality!

Demonstrations at times took the form of disparaging the country and its foundation. Instead of pursuing peaceful avenues for such concerns, protestors often pursued destructive paths, unaware of who was really pulling their strings.

## *The Dumpty falls*

"We have a new way can't you see"
"This country means not much to me"
"Your flag we'll strip from mast above"
"That represents the land you love"
"We have the right to so destroy"
"With methods that we do employ"
But weakened children little know
Who really pulls their strings below
Like Humpty Dumpty on the wall
When strings get pulled, watch Dumpty fall

Protestors continued to roam the streets with placards and signs, "The other side was to blame, Red was to blame, White was to blame, Blue was to blame." What about Scarlet?

## *Lest we should faint*

As much confusion gripped the land
A message from within the band
Of demonstrators all around
Who roamed the streets from town to town
With signs and placards to proclaim
The other side it was to blame
Yet this upheaval we all knew
Was rampant through the Red and Blue
But now and then as was the case
With such unfailing love and grace
A mural seen with Scarlet paint
"In God we trust" …lest we should faint

Unfortunately, many innocent people were injured seriously while mobs pillaged property and businesses during many violent demonstrations.

## *Old Pete*

Old Pete went to the store one day
Not knowing mob was there to play
Just needed milk, and eggs, and bread
But waiting on the streets instead
Was angry crowd outside the store
With brick in hand, and rage galore
While simply shopping in the place
This brick then came to Old Pete's face
A nice old man his price to pay
Just needed food that rainy day
A kind old man nobody knew
Just went to store to get a few

The Declaration of Independence was adopted by the Second Continental Congress on July 4,1776 in Philadelphia, Pennsylvania. It was the first formal statement by our nation asserting the people's right to choose their government. For over 200 years, it has been one of the pillars of our nations strength and resolve.

## *The Declaration*

A faded parchment not worth much?
By men so deeply out of touch
In funny wigs and fancy lace
On Pennsylvania's hallowed place
A "Declaration" was its name
By "Divine" wisdom they proclaim
A Declaration from the dust
All based on what, "In God we trust?"
I'd rather tear down statues tall
And cheer as they begin to fall
So now you ask the reason why?
"My inner rage to satisfy!"

Random crime, shootings and lawlessness continued in major cities across the country throughout 2020, 2021, and well into 2022. Often, innocent bystanders and young children were the victims of such violence.

## *I was only eight*

Was only eight that sunny day
When in my yard went out to play
Then Mommy said we had to go
To market for some stuff you know
So on the bus and into town
As I began to look around
Then painted on the street below
This BLM I didn't know
"Oh Mommy, Mommy, what's this mean?"
"For us my child, to so esteem"
So off the bus into the mall
As came this pain I do recall
"Oh Mommy it does hurt so much"
As felt my Mommy's tender touch
Then in a place with Golden Street
A man all dressed in white to meet
"You now are safe my little child"
I looked at him… and then I smiled

Shootings at times were often directed at those along the "Thin Blue Line." Numerous dedicated police officers across the country lost their lives to criminals and thugs who specifically singled them out for their wanton violence.

## *While on the beat*

On duty one night on the beat
While City sweltered in the heat
A boy came up to ask of me
For help and maybe some money
He seemed so friendly and so kind
So thought I'd help as was inclined
Then reaching in my jacket pock
A shot rang out from young boy's Glock
The Doctors and the Nurses here
To help as they are ever near
This pain and anguish now the price
For trying simply to be nice

# KENOSHA

During August of 2020, unrest and violence erupted in the city of Kenosha, Wisconsin as a result of the police shooting of Jacob Blake. Seventeen year old Kyle Rittenhouse traveled to Kenosha from Antioch, Illinois ( approximately 25 miles away ) to help protect peoples property during the demonstrations. He obtained an AR-15 rifle from a friend who apparently purchased it in Wisconsin.

On the evening of August 25, 2020, while on the streets in Kenosha, Kyle was attacked by several people in the angry mob. He protected himself by killing two of his attackers with his AR-15 and injuring another. Kyle was charged with several serious felony offenses. His defense was that he had a right under the law to defend himself since he felt his life was threatened. The jury upheld his position, finding him not guilty on all charges.

So a guy named Kyle Rittenhouse decided to go to Kenosha, Wisconsin one day to help protect the property and person of those affected by the riots there.

## *Kenosha Kyle*

So one day Kyle decided to
Go to Kenosha…help a few
Got in his car and took the trip
Then put AR upon his hip
In "Badger" land he looked around
And saw the mobs all through the town
He tried to help as best he could
To do the things he thought he should
But some did not accept his plan
And so attacked him as he ran
Then three crazed hoodlums separately
To take his life as he did flee
And one by one his AR fired
Two of the three were then retired
So then young Kyle to jail he went
Five days the jury then was spent
To reach a verdict was their course
His right to use such deadly force
Not guilty they did so decree
As Kyle in court fell to his knee
So what's the motto of this rhyme?
Defend yourself…it's not a crime!

# *MEXICO BORDER CRISIS*

During the years President Donald Trump was in office, our southern border with Mexico was made more secure by building a wall and instituting certain restrictions affecting those coming into our country. Prior to being elected, Joe Biden ran on a platform of dismantling the wall and making our southern border more accessible. Upon being elected President, he did just that. The result was chaos.

Both Vice President Kamala Harris and Homeland Security Secretary Alejandro Mayorkas were delegated the responsibility of managing the crisis. Neither had any significant impact on resolving the issue.

*J. Michael Orr*

Once elected, President Joe Biden kept his promise. He instituted an "Open Door" policy at the US / Mexico border and ceased building the wall. The result was chaos! So why did he do it?

## *No need to fret*

Our borders they are open wide
Seems nothing left to stem the tide
Come one and all cross Rio Grande
To milk and honey fairyland
For healthy care and money free
So very safe you'll always be
No need to grieve, no need to pay
In nice hotels we'll let you stay
But now new message in the air
From guy in White House over there
"The rooms are full, no vacancy!"
"I've changed my mind, can't think you see"
"So give me time, I need a break"
"Back in my room, a nap to take"
"We'll let Kamala take the lead"
But she says, "No, I do not need!"
So young boys sprawled upon the floor
All due to White House open door
But then again no need to fret
The gangs are waiting… unloved pet

Early in his presidency, Joe Biden was rarely seen by the American public. He refused to hold open press conferences, often receiving widespread criticism for his aloofness and secluded manner of behavior, especially when confronted about his position regarding the southern border.

## *Oh sleepy Joe*

Joe Biden says he has a plan
To fix the border if he can
But in the basement now asleep
He snores away without a peep
Then out he comes from hibernate
To speak to us, we cannot wait
"What is your plan oh sleepy Joe?"
"We're so confused and want to know"
"I'll make it clear, and then you'll clap"
"But as for now…I need a nap!"

Joe Biden has always been a career politician. He's never held a real job, never had to make a payroll. Yet simply as a politician all his life, he's managed to amass a net worth estimated in the millions. Not bad for someone who can't even remember where he is half the time and stumbles through most presentations when he steps to the podium. So come on out Joe. We've got some questions to ask!

## *"Come on man!"*

A guy some time ago became
A senator now in the game
He took an oath on bended knee
So young a man and ripe was he
For forty-eight all through the day
He worked at it and got his pay
No other job he ever knew
But millions over in his shoe
Now President of all the land
The worlds destruction in his hand
"So where've you been oh sleepy Joe?"
"There's many things we need to know"
"Why did you open borders wide?"
"This Waterloo now quick to ride"
"Across our country hurting so"
"From pain already, don't you know?"
"So come on out, hey come on man!"
"And answer questions…if you can?"

# AFGHANISTAN WITHDRAWAL

The War in Afghanistan began in 2001 after the September 11 attacks on the World Trade Centers in New York City. It lasted more than 19 years, making it the longest conflict in which the United States had been involved. President Joe Biden felt the war in Afghanistan was never meant to be a long one. He officially announced the withdrawal of the remaining 2,500 United States troops in the country beginning May 1, 2021, to be concluded by September 11, 2021, the anniversary of the war. The only problem was "how" President Joe Biden did it.

The withdrawal of American troops was a debacle of epoch proportions, leaving many of our citizens and Afghani supporters behind in addition to millions of dollars in vital equipment the Taliban quickly confiscated. In addition, thirteen United States men and woman service personnel lost their lives to a suicide bomber while they were protecting and helping those at Kabul's international airport.

On August 29, 2021, the thirteen dead US service members were returned to Dover Air Force Base, Delaware in flag-draped transfer cases. President Joe Biden and his wife were in attendance. While the coffins were being removed from the plane, in an awkward insensitive moment caught on tape, President Joe was seen "checking his watch." Musta had something more important to do at the time.

On May 1, 2021, President Biden ordered the complete withdrawal of troops from Afghanistan. It was a debacle of epoch proportions.

# *It's just my style*

So Joe said we should leave that place
No longer country to embrace
The land they call Afghanistan
Now ruled by heartless Taliban
So leave the stuff and arms behind
No need to fret, we must be kind
So billions strong and loot galore
For Taliban to wage its war
"But what about those left behind?"
"The ones you said you could not find?"
"How come you messed this up sir Joe?"
"It's just my style, did not you know?"

On August 29, 2021, thirteen dead US service members killed during the Afghanistan withdrawal were returned to Dover Air Force Base, Delaware in flag-draped transfer cases while Joe stood by and checked his watch.

## *Coffins off the plane*

So now the mighty USA
Has Taliban the price to pay
They spit on us, and act so tough
While Joe then leaves them all our stuff
These vermin should receive just due
But Joe seems not to have a clue
He talks the talk, but not the walk
And what he says is mostly crock
While coffins did come off the plane
He checked his watch to much disdain!
Who does he think that he must be?
King of the crown with only key?
Oh Joe, you need to listen to
Those with the wisdom more than you

# *HOMELESSNESS*

Throughout 2020, 2021, and well into 2022, homelessness continued to be a major problem in the country. There seemed to be no end in site to this tragic dilemma. An estimated 17 people per 10,000 become homeless each day. In 2021, there were approximately 550,000 homeless in the United States, 13,000 added each year. The life expectancy of a homeless person was 50 years.

Homelessness occurs in most major cities. However, it could not be more evident in places such as Los Angeles and San Francisco, resulting in wide spread use of drugs, crime, and squalor. San Francisco alone had an estimated 5000 homeless persons living in camps across the city in 2021, and more to be expected in 2022.

The "City by the Golden Gate," once known as the "Paris of the West," appears to be losing its dazzle as an alluring destination due to the effects of homelessness. As a result, many of its long term residents have left, seeking other more palatable domains.

Of San Francisco's thousands of people who are currently unhoused, over 70 percent are "unsheltered." They sleep out of doors, in tents, and under highway overpasses.

## *"Un"Golden Gate*

A dark conundrum now at hand
That spans our country's beauty land
And peers down on the camps below
As empty needles ebb and flow
Through Golden Gate that brightly stood
But now in ruins that neighborhood
Where scores now lie in bitter cold
Across the park five-thousand fold
With signs and placards they do plea
For help and some security
"We need a place that we can find"
"For us and pets to just unwind"

# *CANCEL CULTURE*

Cancel culture or "Call-out culture" is a modern form of ostracism in which someone is thrust out of social or professional circles, whether it be online, on social media, or in person. Those subject to this ostracism have been said to be "cancelled." The expression "Cancel Culture" has mostly negative connotations and is used in debates on free speech and censorship.

In addition, the "Cancel Culture" movement at times seeks to inject into the education system of local communities curriculums that often go contrary to accepted norms of education. These positions by school Boards and educators may offend parents and interfere with their right to have input regarding the education of their children.

Woke-ness ~ Political Correctness ~ Do this ~ Don't do that ~ Teach this to our children ~ Don't teach that ~ Tear down this ~ Tear down that.........on and on!

Parents across the country have become outraged at what teachers are teaching their young children, often confronting school boards regarding this sensitive matter.

## *Just a myth*

"Good morning, I'm his teacher here"
"You're little boy, he seems so dear"
"We'll see you back at three o'clock"
"Now Billy dear let's take a walk"
"Down to the classroom where you will meet"
"The other boys and girls so sweet"
"Good morning all, I have a treat"
"Here's Billy Bob for you to meet"
"Now take your seats and we'll begin"
"To talk about our lost nation"
"And crazies who believe in God"
"With family values very odd"
"Yes, Billy did you want to speak?"
"Now from your little boyhood cheek?"
"Yes teacher, I just had a thought"
"About a question that I ought"
"Where's read'n, write'n, and arith?"
"Oh Billy dear, that's just a myth"

This "Cancel Culture" thing has really gotten out of hand. Last week my local Home Owners Association enacted a new amendment to our CC&R's. We're now only allowed "Two Farts" if we need to pass gas!

## *Two farts only ~ The "New Code"*

This "Cancel Culture" in the air
A bit too much for me to bear
They don't like this, they don't like that
Who cares you looney bureaucrat
And now I'm told so many farts
That I'm allowed before I start
To blast my gas within the air
While lady by me starts to glare
"What is this now…two farts by code?"
"Man I need five…or I'll explode!"

# MISS "MURDER HORNET"

The "Murder Hornet" is the world's largest hornet of Asian decent. In December of 2019, "Murder Hornets" were first detected on a highway in Washington State. They arrived by cargo ship. By May 2020, one queen "Murder Hornet" was breeding. The need to eradicate them quickly was evident. The main risk was to our bee population, especially true of "social" types of bees that live in hives and make honey. The hornets attack in late summer and fall when worker hornets need to provide food for developing young. They attack the beehive, kill adult bees, leave their bodies, then take developing bees in the form of larvae and pupae back to their nests for food.

"Murder Hornets" aren't usually aggressive to humans. But they will sting to protect their nest or to keep you away from a beehive they've invaded. If that happens, their larger size sting is worse than other insects. The stinger is longer than that of other wasps and can deliver much more venom and damage tissue. "Murder Hornets" can sting several times. Though it's very rare for a group of hornets to attack a human, it can be very serious if it does occur.

Sometime late in 2019, a few huge "Murder Hornets" took a hike on a cargo ship from somewhere in the orient. The ship landed on the coast of Washington State where the hornets quickly exited the ship looking for a new B & B.

## *What is her name?*

The ship was moored upon the dock
As happy throng came down catwalk
Then flew this lovely off the boat,
All dressed in graceful stylish coat
Of black and orange stately queen
A thing of beauty rarely seen
She flies off quickly with her mate
In Husky State to propagate
With noble skill and grace sublime
She plants her young in overtime
Then off to find another knave
To so become a willing slave
Take care not to offend this dame
Miss "Murder Hornet"…is  her name!

The COVID virus curve seemed to be moving down in the summer of 2021. Things appeared to be getting back to normal, especially up at a local golf course in the state of Washington. So some golfing buddies set up a tee time, got their sticks, and headed to the links.

## *"What the hell is that!"*

We're told the curve is moving down
The scourge that came from Wuhan town
So on the golf course here we go
With drinks in hand and clubs in tow
We've reached the green, I'm now away
So grab my putter, I'm set to play
With steadfast hands, I let it roll
It takes the break, then in the hole
I reach down in to take it out
Then quickly back with horror shout
"What is that thing down in there lies?"
With evil eyes now off it fly's
To darkened forest very near
As our brave foursome starts to fear
This new found thing that comes in spades
The "Murder Hornet"... now invades

# *CALIFORNIA*

For years, millions migrated to the Golden State for a piece of the American dream. The warm weather, beaches, opportunities, laid back life style, cleanliness, and all the rest the state offered attracted multitudes. Now people are leaving the "Golden" state. It seems the gold has rusted a bit. Bad government, highest sales tax rate in the country, second highest gas tax, highest "under" employment rate, California high school students rank 46th in math and 49th in reading, twice the debt as other states, worst health care system in the country, highest poverty rate in the nation, operating costs for businesses 23% higher than the national average, horrible traffic, and Los Angeles is now considered to be the "Gang Capitol" of America......plus more!

The lyrics of an old Golden State song go like this:

"California here I come, right back where I started from. Where bowers of flowers bloom in the sun. Each morning at dawning, birdies sing an' everything. A Sunkist miss said, "Don't be late" that's why I can hardly wait. Open up that Golden Gate, California here I come."

Heard the lyrics of the new state song?

"California here I go...got to find a new pueblo!"

"Margie, ......I think its time to leave the Golden State."

## *"EAST we go"*

A beck and call from Golden State
A place away from winters fate
The warmth, the ocean's beauty surf
A journey long but was the worth
Such effort took to reach this place
But now we pack and join the race
With others going anywhere
Away from all the bleak despair
We stayed for oh so very long
A place we felt we did belong
But now no longer can we bear
The squalor that seems everywhere
In neighborhoods and on our street
We strived so much to keep it neat
Was once we said,"It's Westward Ho!"
In SUV now "EAST we go!"

California recorded its largest fire season ever in 2020. Five of the 10 largest wildfires in state history occurred in 2020, including the August Complex fire, which topped the list as the first California wildfire to burn over 1 million acres. The Dixie fire was one of the states largest in history.

## *California ash*

The smoke it would not go away
From Golden State most every day
Our eyes they burned, our throats so sore
Could not go out to play no more
Each day we woke and looked outside
And there it was, both far and wide
They said the rain it soon might come
To calm this angry maelstrom
But ash continued from the sky
To fall on us, both you and I
A holocaust that had been cast
Upon us all…so long would last

The Orange County, California oil spill on October 1, 2021, deposited crude onto popular Southern California beaches. Commercial divers found the pipeline had been displaced with a 13-inch split along the length of the pipe. Investigators suspect that a large container ship dragged its anchor in the area during heavy winds, causing the break.

## *California Oil Spill - October 1, 2021*

October 1, the pipe did pop
One hundred feet below the top
A blackened slick began to dance
Toward southern shores a wide expanse
The beaches now the experts say
A heavy price they soon would pay
On ocean's floor the oil did leak
Now south beach land so ever bleak
Another wound on Golden State
October 1, that was the date

# *EVERYDAY STUFF*

You need to make an important phone call, and must actually "talk" with someone. So you dial it up, then the recording says, "Please excuse us, but we're experiencing a high volume of calls." A "high volume" of calls at 3:00 am in the morning? Give me a break! So now you're placed on hold listening to music you'd rather not. Then, just when it seems you're about to connect, another message comes on, causing you to pull out your hair, if you've got any left! You've already been waiting 10 minutes. Now you get disconnected!

Some of you may be old enough to remember the days when you made a phone call and an actual "live person" answered the phone. What a novelty!

"Please excuse us. We're experiencing a high volume of calls."

## *You are caller 9*

I need to put my mind at ease
And wish to talk with someone please
Recording says I'm caller 5
"You'll soon connect with agent live"
"But as for now please do enjoy"
"This loud punk music we employ"
So now with patience here I wait
"Be with you soon, now caller 8"
But I thought I was caller 5?
To speak with someone who's alive
This waiting really gets to me
I've things to do, I've got to pee
"Oh hello sir, could you please hold?"
"You're caller 9"…now I am told!

# *OLD AGE*

Many of you may be in the "Old Age" category. Old Age has been defined as ages nearing or surpassing the life expectancy of human beings, and is thus the end of the human life cycle. So what does this mean? It was once felt when you hit the age of 65 you were "old," which meant you started to receive Medicare and retired from your job. However, people are now generally living longer lives. Either way, old age comes with a price.

If you're old like me, you've probably experienced some of these things. Spending half your life in Dr.'s offices, sorting out your medications daily to make certain you take your blood thinner instead of a stool softener, getting up five times a night to pee, having difficulty getting out of bed and putting on your clothes, watching every step you take to make sure you don't trip and break your neck, or trying to do things your mind wants to do but your body doesn't. In addition, you may have some form of disability like me. One of the Rhymes on the following pages, *Lost brother dear,* addresses my being born blind in one eye, having only one good eye. Always something huh?

As older persons, we often recall when times were much simpler, drifting back in our thoughts to those days and places we once knew. Maybe we even go back and visit them now and then.

I was once able to hit the ball off the tee 300 yards. Now I can barely crank it 150. It takes me forever to get dressed in the morning and I've got to watch every step I take to make sure I don't fall and break my neck. Spend half my time in Dr's offices and know most of the other patients there. Feels like I'm back in traffic school. Old age sucks !

## *Mind go, body no*

I'm not the same today you see
Once young, and strong, and filled with glee
Now frail this body hurts within
My mind says go, but body thin
I beckon youth to no avail
A simple spark to split the rail
This frame now battles pain's halo
My mind says go…my body no

The other day, my wife reminded me I had a Dental appointment on Thursday morning. My response, "I have a Dentist?" Like I said, old age can suck at times!

## *I've now got to pee!*

I'm big in the middle
Small at the top
My teeth keep on hurting
They're starting to drop
So hard in the morning
To get out of bed
Then into the bathroom
I feel like I'm dead
Now down to the kitchen
With splitting headache
The walk is so hard
How long will it take
With coffee in hand
Now on with TV
Then wouldn't you know, I've now got to pee!

Any of you reading this on Diuretic medication? If so, you might be able to relate to this. So my wife and I are driving down the highway and all of a sudden I've got to pee. Can't hold it any longer. No gas station in sight and no tree's either. What to do? Stop, park on the side of the highway, get out of the car.....and pee! I now need to pee so much at night that I have a bottle next to my bed so I don't need to get up! Sound familiar?

## Six times a night

I'm up six times a night to pee
This lack of sleep not good for me
When I was young, was just a few
And now and then to take a poo
So now this bottle by my bed
Then back to bed you sleepy head
You laugh at me, best listen friend
This is what happens near the end!

So now they say you're a "Pre Diabetic." The tests also show you're starting to rust around the edges. The Doctor tells you it might be a good idea to make an appointment at a local body shop to get some repairs done.

## *Don't want to fall*

Pre Diabetic I am told
Another thing now that I'm old
The lab tests say I'm not so great
They tell me that I must lose weight
The pills stacked neatly in a row
As pharmacies take all my dough
So now its bad cholesterol
And be alert, don't want to fall
So then I'm told more pills to trust
To fix this frame, that's gone to rust!

So you're strong, work out every day, lift those weights, watch your diet, do everything needed. Life is good right? Old age, a cane, a walker, leg cramps at night. Not on your day timer huh?

## *Someday you'll know*

These cramps they never go away
It seems I have them everyday
They mostly come while I'm asleep
Then like a rocket out I leap
Upon the nearby waiting floor
Then quickly to the bathroom door
Where now I need to take a pee
While cramps continue down my knee
I can't remember so much fun
As down my leg the pain does run
You think its funny now you say?
Someday you'll know…as you decay!

The author, J. Michael Orr, was born with only one good eye, a congenital defect at birth. Although his left eye had some limited peripheral vision, old age eventually took its toll, rendering the left eye completely blind.

## *Lost brother dear*

Out of the womb, one eye to use
A tragedy I did not choose
This message to my mother came
"Oh mother dear you weren't to blame"
So through the years one beacon strong
While other scantly came along
Beside the one that was so bright
To navigate throughout the night
Then on one day my brother found
A darkened place that did abound
With deep abyss and no way out
As came a mournful sombre shout
"I must now leave you brother dear"
"My failing lamp is out I fear"
Back on the path, one beacon strong
No brother dear to come along

Often, we recall when times were much simpler, drifting back in our thoughts to those days and places we once knew. Maybe even going back to visit them now and then.

## *The place I knew*

I took a trip one day to see
The neighborhood that nurtured me
In olden days the house I had
Now changed so much and over clad
With scrub and thickets on its face
So many things now out of place
Yet even though the home I knew
Where I was raised and wholesome grew
Is now a relic changed so much
Still in my mind I stay in touch
And now and then I go to see
The neighborhood that nurtured me

# THE FINAL RHYME

In December 2021 I finished the 81st rhyme, my age at the time. Then, at the end of 2021 when we all thought COVID-19 was beginning to wane a bit, a new visitor got off the bus at dawn one morning.

## *81 rhymes I did write*

A while ago when I was young
Began to scribe til I was done
Then 81 did I so write
Amongst pandemics daily fight
Who could have known the grievous times
That gave me pause to write these rhymes
Now vaccine jab and booster had
To be immune, to make me glad
So what to do now that I'm done?
Enjoy a beer and have some fun
But who is that just off the bus?
To hassle and to bother us?
Who is that brat arrived at dawn?
"I think they call him Omicron"

So here we are 2022, what do we now look forward to, the past two years oh such a curse, we pray the next would be less worse

J. Michael Orr

CPSIA information can be obtained
at www.ICGtesting.com
Printed in the USA
BVHW060945150322
631524BV00011B/846